CROHN's DISEASE
FOOD LIST

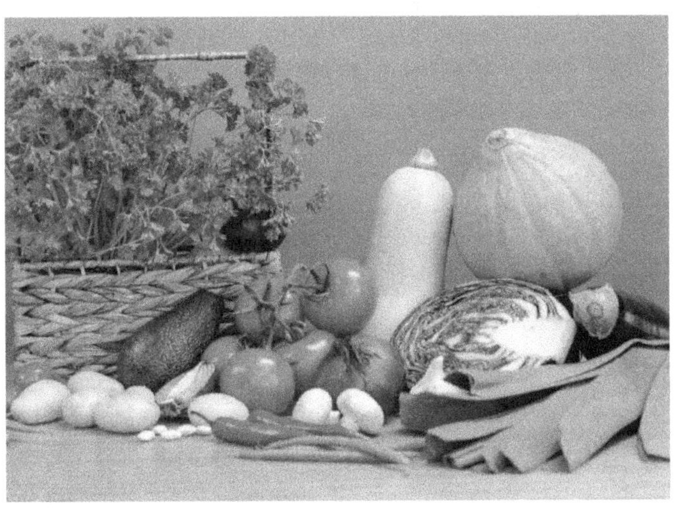

A Comprehensive Guide with Nutritional Guidance to Soothe Your Gut and Foster Overall Well-being

BELL QUINTANA

TABLE OF CONTENT

INTRODUCTION

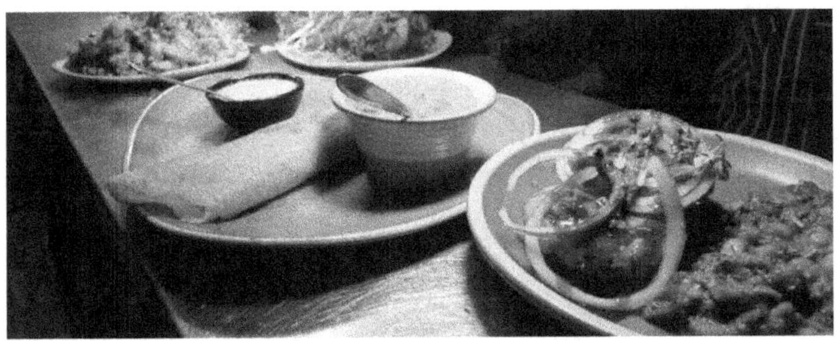

Welcome to "Crohn's Disease Food List"

In the realm of health and nutrition, understanding the intricate dance between what we consume and our body's response is crucial. This book is a tailored guide designed to empower individuals navigating the complexities of Crohn's disease through the lens of nutrition.

Crohn's disease, an inflammatory bowel condition, is a formidable adversary that affects millions worldwide. It presents a unique set of challenges, often influencing not only physical health but also the delicate balance of daily life. The intricacies of Crohn's are like a puzzle, with each person's experience being a distinctive piece. To unravel this mystery, we delve into the profound connection between diet and the management of Crohn's disease.

Why This Book Matters

As a seasoned health nutritionist, I've witnessed the transformative power of dietary choices on individuals grappling with Crohn's. This book is not just a compilation of food lists; it's a roadmap for nourishing your body, understanding its signals, and embracing a lifestyle that fosters vitality despite the challenges of Crohn's disease.

Within these pages, you'll discover a comprehensive exploration of Crohn's-friendly foods, practical meal planning tips, and expert insights from healthcare professionals and dietitians. Real stories from those who've triumphed over adversity will serve as beacons of inspiration, guiding you through the sometimes tumultuous journey towards wellness.

We'll address the burning questions you may have, debunk misconceptions, and equip you with the tools to confidently navigate grocery aisles, restaurant menus, and social gatherings. This book is not just about adapting your diet; it's about transforming your relationship with food to become an ally in your quest for well-being.

So, embark on this journey with an open mind and a willingness to embrace change. The path to managing Crohn's disease is unique for each individual, and this book is your companion, offering support, knowledge, and a roadmap to rediscover a sense of control over your health.

Let the exploration begin, and may your journey be one of empowerment, resilience, and ultimately, triumph over adversity.

Understanding Crohn's Disease

In the symphony of the human body, the gastrointestinal tract plays a pivotal role, orchestrating the complex dance of digestion, absorption, and elimination. Yet, for individuals grappling with Crohn's disease, this harmonious composition is disrupted, and the once melodious notes become a challenging discord.

Crohn's disease, a chronic inflammatory condition, sets the stage for a unique set of challenges within the intricate landscape of the digestive system. Imagine your digestive tract as a finely tuned instrument, and Crohn's as a rogue musician disrupting the rhythm. The result: inflammation, discomfort, and a cascade of symptoms that extend beyond the digestive realm.

At the heart of Crohn's lies an overactive immune system. Picture your immune system as a vigilant guardian, defending your body against invaders. In Crohn's disease, this vigilant guardian turns on its host, mistaking the lining of the digestive tract for a threat. This relentless assault triggers inflammation, leading to the hallmark symptoms of Crohn's, including abdominal pain, diarrhea, fatigue, and weight loss.

While the primary battleground of Crohn's is the gastrointestinal tract, its influence extends far beyond. The systemic nature of the disease can affect joints, skin, eyes, and even lead to complications such as nutritional deficiencies. Understanding this holistic impact is key to crafting a comprehensive approach to management.

Crohn's disease often has a genetic component, with certain individuals more predisposed to its development. However, genes alone do not tell the full story. Environmental factors, such as diet, lifestyle, and the delicate balance of the gut microbiome, can act as triggers, either igniting or dampening the flames of inflammation.

Diagnosing Crohn's involves a meticulous process that combines clinical evaluation, imaging studies, and sometimes endoscopy. Yet, the road to diagnosis can be winding, with symptoms often mimicking other gastrointestinal conditions. Early detection is paramount, as it allows for timely intervention and management.

Understanding the intricacies of Crohn's disease is not merely an academic pursuit; it is the cornerstone of empowerment for individuals navigating this challenging terrain. Armed with knowledge, individuals can actively participate in their care, make informed decisions, and collaborate effectively with healthcare professionals to sculpt a personalized management plan.

In the chapters that follow, we will embark on a journey of exploration, unraveling the nuances of Crohn's-friendly nutrition, lifestyle choices, and the resilience of the human spirit. Join me as we dive into the heart of the matter, demystifying Crohn's disease, and crafting a symphony of wellness amidst the discord.

CHAPTER 1

FOUNDATION OF CROHN'S-FRIENDLY EATING

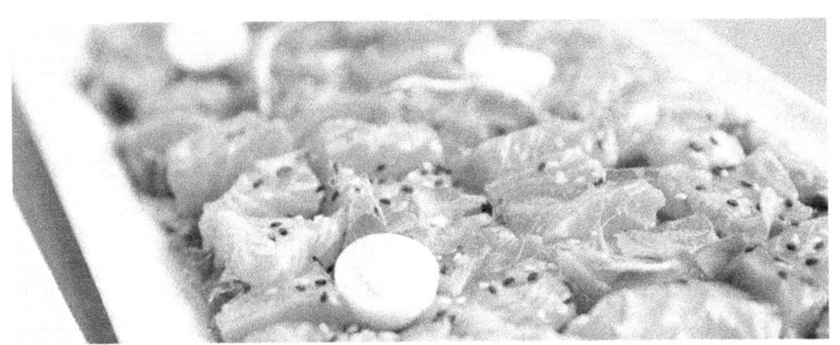

Overview of Crohn's-Friendly Foods

Enter the core of this chapter, where we'll reveal the carefully curated list of Crohn's-friendly foods that are not only helpful in managing symptoms but also serve as allies in your quest for optimal health. This is not just a list; it is a veritable gold mine of nutrient-dense power foods that will fuel your body, calm your digestive tract, and give you more energy in the day-to-day grind.

1. <u>LEAN PROTEINS</u>

Think of lean proteins as the building blocks of your body's toughness. These proteins, which may be found in fish, chicken, eggs, and plant-based foods like tofu and lentils, provide your foundation for strength. Packed with vital amino acids, they promote muscular health, facilitate tissue healing, and help maintain a steady level of energy. Learn how to balance your sources of protein so that your plate is enriched and your body is strengthened.

2.   LOW-RESIDUE VEGETABLES

Welcome to the world of low-residue veggies, a delicious variety that promises to be kind to your digestive tract. Among your buddies are veggies like spinach, zucchini, carrots, and cucumbers; they provide vital vitamins, minerals, and fiber without overloading your digestive system. Discover the skill of cooking these veggies so they become delectable meals that will satisfy your palate and nourish your health.

3.   BERRIES AND FRUITS

Explore the colorful world of fruits and berries, the delightful nutritional symphony of nature. These fruits, which range from oranges to papayas, blueberries to bananas, are naturally sweet and packed with vitamins and antioxidants. Find the best times and combinations to improve the fruit's digestion, so it becomes a tasty and nourishing complement to your regular meals.

4.   STARCHES AND GRAINS

Starches and grains are essential for maintaining your energy stores. Your partners in delivering complex carbs that release energy continuously throughout the day include quinoa, rice, sweet potatoes, and oats. Discover the art of cooking by transforming these staples into filling, healthy meals that meet your body's energy requirements without causing inflammation.

Every component in this Crohn's-friendly food excursion is a gem, carefully selected to offer not just nourishment but also a symphony of nutrients that enhance your general health. As we progress through this chapter, remember the significance of every dietary decision and the possibility of nourishment that goes well beyond treating symptoms.

Your plate is a palette of colorful, health-promoting options rather than just a blank canvas. Allow these meals to be your allies as you strive for a robust and vibrant existence.

Importance of Nutritional Balance

Nutrition is about the harmony that the various foods on your plate make within your body, not just the individual foods. Maintaining proper vitamin and mineral levels, managing your hydration, and balancing your macronutrient intake are all essential for bolstering your body's resistance to Crohn's disease. This section will assist you in creating meals that are in balance with your body's requirements.

Listening to Your Body's Signals

Your body is an amazing communicator; it frequently gives you tiny hints about what it needs. When it comes to Crohn's-friendly nutrition, it's critical to recognise these cues. We dive into the practice of mindful eating, examining how it may be a valuable tool in your toolbox to pay attention to your body's signals about hunger, fullness, and how it reacts to certain foods.

As we delve further into this chapter, remember that the foundation we are laying is about abundance through wise decision-making, not just limitation. This is an adventure, a quest to find meals that enhance your dining experience while simultaneously providing your body with nourishment.

We'll go into the specifics of Crohn's-safe meals in the upcoming sections, giving you a thorough guide to help you load your plate with healthy options. Together, let's set out on this path to create a foundation that enables your nutritional decisions to be in line with your innate resilience.

CHAPTER 2

CROHN'S-SAFE FOODS

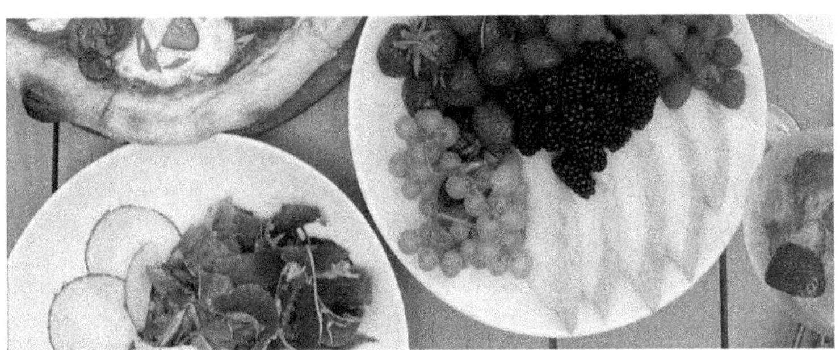

Welcome to Chapter 2, this chapter explores Crohn's-safe meals, which have been carefully chosen to be both transformative in terms of their nutritional power and easy on your digestive system. Consider this to be your culinary compass, pointing you in the direction of a landscape where resilience and nourishment coexist.

HIGH-NUTRIENT, LOW-IRRITATION CHOICES

The arrangement of your plate plays a crucial role in the symphony of Crohn's disease-friendly dining. Here, we break down the nuances of high-nutrient, low-irritation options—a decision that isn't only based on flavor, but also thoughtfully designed to nourish your body and be kind to your digestive system.

Lean Proteins: The Backbone of Resilience

Your dietary resiliency is anchored by lean proteins. These proteins, which are high in vital amino acids, are the building blocks your body needs to maintain healthy muscles and repair damaged tissue. Go for foods like fish, eggs, skinless chicken, and plant-based foods like lentils and tofu. Making informed choices guarantees that your body gets the essential nutrients it needs to function and gives you long-lasting energy without causing inflammation. Here's a detailed list of lean proteins along with their nutritional values to help you on your path to health:

1. SKINLESS POULTRY:

Cooked, skinless chicken breast:

Nutritional information:

- 31g of protein per 100g
- 165 calories per 100 grammes
- 3.6g of fat per 100g
- High in phosphorus, selenium, vitamin B6, and niacin.

Skinless, roasted turkey breast:

<u>Nutritional information:</u>

- 29g of protein per 100g
- 135 calories per 100 grammes
- One gramme of fat for every 100 grammes
- Good source of phosphorus, vitamin B6, niacin, and protein.

Baked or grilled salmon:

<u>Nutritional information:</u>

- 25g of protein per 100g
- 206 calories per 100 grammes
- Selenium, vitamin B12, vitamin D, and omega-3 fatty acids are all in large amounts.

Cod (grilled or baked):

<u>Nutritional information:</u>

- 20g of protein per 100g
- 100g has 105 calories.
- Low in fat and a great source of vitamin B12 and phosphorus.

2. EGGS:

Boiled or scrambled egg whites:

Nutritional information:

- 11g of protein per 100g
- 52 calories per 100 grammes
- High in protein, practically fat-free, and a good source of selenium.

Whole eggs, either poached or boiled:

Nutritional information:

- 13g of protein per 100g
- 100g has 155 calories.
- Rich in choline, biotin, and other micronutrients.

3. PLANT-BASED SOLUTIONS:

Firm, cooked tofu:

Nutritional information:

- Protein (g/100g): 15g
- 100g has 144 calories.
- Excellent supply of magnesium, calcium, and iron.

Cooked lentils:

Nutritional information:

- 9g of protein per 100g
- 100g has 116 calories.
- Rich in manganese, iron, folate, and fibre.

Cooked chickpeas:

Nutritional information:

- 8.9g of protein per 100g
- 100g has 164 calories.
- Packed with vitamins, fiber, folate, and manganese.

4. ALTERNATIVES TO LEAN MEAT:

- Grilled or baked sausages made of turkey or chicken:
- Protein: Depending on the brand, usually 12–15 grams per serving.
- Verify the nutritional data for a particular product.
- Seek for low-fat products with less ingredients.

Note: Due to differences in product brands and cooking techniques, nutritional information is approximate and subject to change. For individualized guidance, always refer to the packaging and speak with a medical practitioner or dietician.

To guarantee a well-rounded nutritional profile, think about combining a variety of these lean protein options as you investigate them. Try a variety of cooking techniques and flavor combinations to ensure that your meals are not only filling but also delightful. Bon appétit to the core of your resiliency!

Key Takeaways:

1. Spread out your sources of protein to get the most nutritious value.
2. For variation, try to find lean cuts and investigate plant-based protein sources.
3. Give preference to cooking techniques that are easy on the digestive tract, such steaming, grilling, or baking.

Low-Residue Vegetables: A Garden of Gentle Delights

Step into the world of low-residue veggies, a garden of mild pleasures that will soothe your palate and promote intestinal balance at the same time. Consider vegetables like spinach, zucchini, carrots and cucumbers—each one selected for its high nutrient content and low gastrointestinal distress. Packed in fiber, vitamins, and minerals, these veggies support general health without taxing the body. Below is an extensive list of low-residue veggies together with their nutritional values to help you on your journey to health:

1. LEAFY GREENS:

Sautéed or steamed spinach:

Nutritional information:

- 2.2g of fiber per 100g
- 23 calories per 100 grammes
- High in iron, folate, vitamin A, and vitamin K.

Romaine Lettuce(Raw):

Nutritional information:

- 1.2g of fiber per 100g
- 17 calories per 100 grammes
- Excellent source of folate, vitamin K, and C.

2. ZUCCHINI:

Zucchini (cooked or grilled):

Nutritional information:

- One gramme of fiber for every 100 grammes
- 17 calories per 100 grammes
- Contains potassium, vitamin B6, and vitamin C.

3. CARROTS:

Pureed or cooked carrots:

Nutritional information:

- 2.8g of fiber per 100g
- 41 calories per 100 grammes
- High in potassium, vitamin K, and beta-carotene.

4. CUCUMBERS:

Pickled or raw cucumbers:

Nutritional information:

- Fiber content: 0.5g/100g
- 16 calories per 100 grammes
- Potassium and vitamin K-rich, and hydrating.

5. BELL PEPPERS:

Roasted or uncooked bell peppers:

Nutritional information:

- 2.1g of fiber per 100g
- 31 calories per 100 grammes
- Rich in antioxidants, vitamin C, and vitamin A.

6. GREEN BEANS:

Green Beans (steamed or sautéed):

Nutritional information:

- 2.7g of fiber per 100g
- 31 calories per 100 grammes
- Excellent supply of folate, vitamin K, and C.

7. AUBERGINE

Baked or grilled aubergine:

Nutritional information:

- 3g of fiber for every 100g
- 25 calories per 100 grammes
- Has potassium and antioxidants.

Note: Due to differences in product brands and cooking techniques, nutritional information is approximate and subject to change. For individualized guidance, always refer to the packaging and speak with a medical practitioner or dietician.

These low-residue veggies have a mild flavor profile and provide you with the nutrients you need to be healthy. As you look through these choices, think about experimenting with different cooking methods and combos to produce dishes that are satisfying and entertaining.

1. To improve digestion, use veggies that are well-cooked or pureed.
2. Try a variety of preparation techniques, including sautéing or roasting, to see which one works best for your digestive system.
3. To increase the variety of nutrients in your diet, gradually include different kinds of low-residue veggies.

Fruits and Berries: Nature's Nutrient-Rich Jewels

Explore the colorful world of fruits and berries, the nutrient-dense jewels of nature that add flavor and health advantages to your dish. Without upsetting the stomach, bananas, blueberries, oranges, and papayas provide a range of vitamins, antioxidants, and natural sweetness. For maximum enjoyment and nutritional impact, learn to balance your fruit intake by taking ripeness and paring options into consideration. Here's a long list of fruits and berries together with their nutritional values to help you reach a symphony of taste and health:

1. BANANAS:

Ripe banana:

Nutritional information:

- 2.6g of fiber per 100g
- 89 calories per 100 grammes
- Packed with potassium, B6, and C vitamins.

2. BLUEBERRIES:

Frozen or fresh blueberries:

Nutritional information:

- 2.4g of fiber per 100g
- 57 calories per 100 grammes
- Rich in manganese, vitamin C, and antioxidants.

3. ORANGES:

Orange juice, either raw or fresh:

Nutritional information:

- 2.3g of fiber per 100g
- 43 calories per 100 grammes
- Good source of potassium, vitamin A, and vitamin C.

4. PAPAYAS:

Fresh or blended papaya:

Nutritional information:

- 1.7g of fiber per 100g
- 43 calories per 100 grammes
- High in folate, vitamin A, and C.

5. APPLES:

I. Sliced or apple sauced apple:

Nutritional information:

- 2.4g of fiber per 100g
- 52 calories per 100 grammes
- Contains dietary fiber, vitamin C, and antioxidants.

6. BERRIES:

I. Frozen or fresh strawberries:

Nutritional information:

- Fibre content: 2 grammes par 100 grammes
- 32 calories per 100 grammes

- Rich in antioxidants, manganese, and vitamin C.

7. KIWI:

I. Sliced or pureed kiwi:

Nutritional information:

- 3g of fiber for every 100g
- 61 calories per 100 grammes
- High in dietary fiber, vitamin K, and vitamin C.

Note: Depending on the brand of the product and the freshness of the fruit, nutritional information may differ and is approximate. For individualized guidance, always refer to the packaging and speak with a medical practitioner or dietician.

While you appreciate these jewels of nature, think of putting them in fruit salads or smoothies or just eating them by themselves. These fruits and berries offer a palate of culinary delights in addition to improving your overall health due to their diverse flavors and nutritional value. To a symphony of the wonders of nature - feast and be nourished!

Key Takeaways:

1. Select soft, ripe fruits to facilitate easier digestion.
2. To balance blood sugar levels, try eating fruits together with a supply of protein or healthy fats.
3. Try a variety of fruit combinations to see what works best for your digestion and taste.

Grains and Starches: Sustaining Your Energy Reserves with Elegance

Starches and grains take center stage as the graceful maestros that maintain your energy levels. Your partners in delivering complex carbs that release energy continuously throughout the day include quinoa, rice, sweet potatoes, and oats. These options provide a sense of fullness and satisfaction in addition to richness in nutrients, which is important for people managing the difficulties associated with Crohn's disease.

To help you create a well-rounded and satisfying meal, the following is a detailed list of grains and starches along with their nutritional values:

1. QUINOA:

Cooked quinoa:

- 2.8g of fiber per 100g
- 120 calories per 100 grams.
- A complete protein supply that is high in phosphorus, iron, and magnesium.

2. RICE:

Cooked white rice:

- Fiber content: 0.4g/100g
- 130 calories per 100 grams.
- Enriched with niacin and folate, two B-vitamins.

Coated brown rice:

- 1.8g of fiber per 100g
- 100g has 111 calories.
- Greater amounts of fiber and minerals, such as selenium and manganese.

3. SWEET POTATOES:

Baked or mashed sweet potatoes:

- 3.3g of fiber per 100g
- 86 calories per 100 grammes
- High in potassium, vitamin C, and beta-carotene.

4. OATS:

Cooked rolled oats:

- 2.7g of fiber per 100g
- 71 calories per 100 grammes

- Rich in soluble fiber, which makes you feel full.

5. MILLET:

Cooked millet:

- 31.3g of fiber per 100g
- Calories per 100 grammes: 119
- An excellent supply of manganese, phosphorus, and magnesium.

6. SORGHUM

Cooked sorghum:

- 6.7g of fiber per 100g
- 101 calories per 100 grammes
- Antioxidant-rich and free of gluten.

7. BUCKWHEAT:

Cooked buckwheat:

- 2.7g of fiber per 100g
- 92 calories per 100 grammes
- A high-nutrient alternative that is rich in magnesium and manganese.

Note: Due to differences in product brands and cooking techniques, nutritional information is approximate and subject to change. For individualized guidance, always refer to the packaging and speak with a medical practitioner or dietician.

Try experimenting with various cooking methods and adding diversity to your meals as you learn about and work with grains and starches. These choices contribute to the varied nutrient profile that is vital for your overall health in addition to offering long-lasting energy. Bon appétit to a dish full of refinement and nourishment!

Key Takeaways:

1. Go for grains that are simple to digest, such as quinoa or white rice.
2. For variation, try using different grains like sorghum or millet.
3. Give priority to cooking techniques like soaking or boiling that improve digestibility.

Every meal choice in this investigation of nutrient-dense, low-irritating options is a goldmine of health advantages. When navigating this gastronomic world, keep in mind that decisions you make can have a significant impact on your general well-being in addition to flavor. Your plate is a palette of colorful, health-promoting options rather than just a blank canvas.

To a Plate Full of Purpose

CHAPTER 3

FOODS TO LIMIT OR AVOID

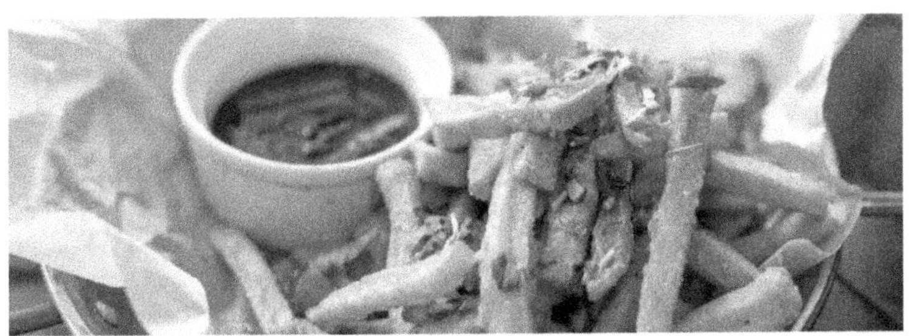

It's critical to understand which meals can worsen symptoms and cause inflammation as we navigate the gastronomic terrain of Crohn's disease management. In-depth discussion of foods to restrict or stay away from is covered in Chapter 3, which will help you navigate the culinary fork in the road with wisdom and purpose.

Trigger Foods and Inflammatory Substances

Here, we look at meals that could serve as triggers, causing inflammation in the sensitive balance of your digestive system. Not only is every option marked for limitation, but it is also thoroughly explained, giving you the ability to make well-informed selections regarding your diet.

✖ HIGH-FAT FOODS:

People with Crohn's disease may find it difficult to consume high-fat foods, even if they are frequently enticing to the palate. They might cause inflammation and add to intestinal irritation.

Restrict or steer clear of:

- ❖ Fried foods (such as fried chicken & French fries)
- ❖ Meats high in fat content, such as processed sausages and high-fat beef
- ❖ dairy items with added fat (whole milk, certain cheeses, etc.)

✖ DAIRY PRODUCTS:

For people with Crohn's disease, dairy products can be controversial, especially if lactose intolerance is an issue.

Exercise caution when dealing with:

- ❖ Whole milk as well as cream
- ❖ Cheeses with a lot of fat
- ❖ Creamy dishes and ice cream

✖ SPICY AND IRRITATING FOODS:

Highly inflammatory foods and spices can cause discomfort and inflammation.

Utilize caution when doing:

- Spicy meals (such as curry and hot peppers)
- Oranges and grapefruits, among other citrus fruits and juices
- Tough-fibered raw veggies, such as raw broccoli and cauliflower

Potential Allergens:

People who have Crohn's disease may be more sensitive to specific allergens, which might worsen their symptoms.

Be careful when dealing with:

- Grains containing gluten, like rye, barley, & wheat
- Certain seafood and shellfish
- Peanuts and tree nuts.

Note: Individual differences may exist in the effects of particular foods. Maintaining a food journal is a good way to pinpoint your own triggers. For individualized guidance, speak with a doctor or dietician.

Consider this chapter as a guide for thoughtful, well-informed decision-making. The intention is to assist your well-being with a conscious attitude, not to impose restrictions just for the purpose of doing so. Cheers to a voyage of well-informed culinary choices and perseverance.

CHAPTER 4

NUTRITIONAL INFORMATION AND MEAL PLANNING

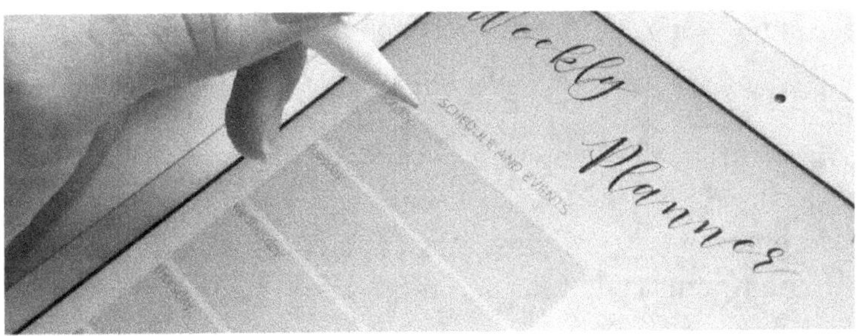

This chapter takes you on a precise journey where meal planning becomes a customised culinary blueprint and nutritional information becomes your compass. It serves as a guide for intentional steps towards well-being through every decision you make, in addition to what's on your plate. Together, we will explore the art and science of creating meals that meet your body's demands and help you achieve maximum health.

Understanding Nutritional Needs

Knowing what your body needs nutritionally is like writing a piece of art in the symphony of wellness—it's distinct, complex, and beautiful. This is not just a list of recommended diets; this is a manual for arranging nutrients into a harmonious whole that complements the unique needs of your body. Let's explore the essential components of comprehending your dietary requirements and creating a unique well-being song.

Individualized Needs for Nutrients

The same way that each instrument in an orchestra needs a particular song, your body has specific nutritional needs as well. These needs are influenced by variables like age, gender, degree of activity, and Crohn's disease demands. A composition that supports your health begins with an understanding of your baseline requirements for macronutrients (proteins, fats, and carbohydrates) and micronutrients (vitamins and minerals).

<u>Advice</u>: Work with a dietitian to customize your nutritional intake according to your unique lifestyle and health profile.

Synergy of Micronutrients

Consider micronutrients as the various instruments in an orchestra, each of which is essential to the composition as a whole. The interplay of these micronutrients is essential for optimum health and resistance to Crohn's disease problems. As an illustration:

Calcium absorption is improved by vitamin D, which is important for healthy bones.

The absorption of nonheme iron from plant-based sources is facilitated by vitamin C.
A balance between zinc and copper promotes immunological activity.
Aim for a colorful, varied dish to organically include a range of micronutrients.

Customising Diet to Address Crohn's Disease Issues

Nutrition can be focused specifically for Crohn's disease patients by acknowledging the unique obstacles this disease presents. For example:

Prioritizing foods that are high in nutrients and readily digested becomes crucial if malabsorption is a concern. Sufficient hydration promotes intestinal health in general and can lessen symptoms like constipation.

Advice: To address the nutritional issues unique to Crohn's disease, collaborate closely with your healthcare team.

The Skill of Intuitive Eating

The art of intuitive eating is like listening to the subtle nuances of your body's cues in the symphony of nutrition. Observe your feelings of hunger, fullness, and how your body reacts to various foods. This attentive approach promotes a healthy connection with food and benefits one's physical and mental health.

<u>**Advice**</u>: Embrace mindful eating by appreciating every taste, paying attention to indications of hunger and fullness, and savoring a range of textures and flavors.

Knowing what kind of food you need is a dynamic process that changes throughout time. It's an exploration of who you are, learning to listen to the harmony of your body's needs and creating meals that fit your own rhythm. We'll turn this knowledge into practical meal planning techniques in the upcoming chapters, pointing you in the direction of a culinary blueprint that complements your path to optimal health. Let the symphony of personalized nutrition begin - to art and science!

Crafting a Crohn's-Friendly Meal Plan

Creating a food plan that works for Crohn's disease is like creating a blueprint for your ideal health. It's not just about what you eat; it's about carefully coordinating your intake of nutrients to meet your body's specific requirements as well as the difficulties that come with having Crohn's disease. Let's examine the essential components of creating a food plan that enhances, sustains, and nourishes your quest for wellbeing.

1. Variety and Balance

Think of your plate as a canvas, and every meal as a unique and well-balanced brushstroke. Aim for a balanced intake of proteins, carbs, and fats as macronutrients to maintain general health and offer long-lasting energy. Add a range of fruits, vegetables, lean meats, and whole grains to create a palette of colors, textures, and flavors.

Advice: In order to guarantee a wide variety of nutrients, follow the "Eat the Rainbow" strategy.

2.   Light Lunches Often

In the realm of Crohn's disease-friendly cuisine, tiny, frequent meals make up a harmonious composition of nourishment. By giving your body a constant supply of nutrients without overburdening your digestive system, this method helps control symptoms. Divide your daily consumption into multiple smaller meals and snacks that are specifically designed to assist and enhance your body's ability to withstand adversity.

<u>Snack ideas:</u> Include protein, good fats, and simple-to-digest carbohydrates.

3.   Conscientious Preparation

One important element in the culinary symphony is the manner you cook your food. Select cooking techniques like baking, steaming, or sautéing that improve digestibility. Try different herbs and spices to enhance flavor without irritating the skin. Carefully preparing your food not only maintains its nutritious value but also makes eating a celebration of well-being.

Try low-residue cooking methods for your veggies to improve their digestibility.

4.   Water

Drinking enough water will help your meal plan's nutritional makeup flow smoothly. Make sure you are drinking enough water, herbal teas, and healthy broths. Drinking enough water aids with digestion, keeps constipation at bay, and promotes gut health in general.

Drink water throughout the day and eat meals high in water content, such as fruits and vegetables, to stay hydrated.

5.   Tracking Initiators

Your body may react differently to different meals, therefore it's important to identify your own triggers in order to create a customized strategy for your diet. Maintain a food journal to monitor your reactions and discover possible triggers. High-fat diets, spicy foods, and some allergies are common triggers.

<u>Advice</u>: Experiment with different foods gradually and see how your body responds.

A meal plan that is Crohn's disease-friendly is not a set recipe; rather, it is a flexible guide that you may modify to suit your changing needs. It's a continuous investigation, a taste adventure that corresponds with the subtleties of your health. Let intention lead your decisions as you plan your meals, and let every mouthful be a note in the harmony of your well-being. Bon appétit to the science and art of preparing wholesome meals!

Breakfast Ideas

Breakfast establishes the tone for your day and provides a chance to start your morning with light food for those with Crohn's disease. The following are some nutrient-dense breakfast suggestions to promote your wellbeing:

1. Breakfast Bowl with Quinoa:
Cooked quinoa with a dollop of Greek yogurt, sliced bananas, and chia seeds on top. This nutritious meal offers probiotics, fiber, and protein in equal measure.

2. Berries with Muesli:
Warm muesli drizzled with honey and adorned with a berry mixture (strawberries, blueberries). Berries contribute natural sweetness and antioxidants, and oats provide soluble fiber for long-lasting energy.

3. Smoothie Bowl:
Add frozen berries, banana, spinach, and a scoop of protein powder to a blender. Add some granola and sliced almonds over top for a filling, high-nutrient start to the day.

4. Toast with egg and avocado:
Avocado slices are served alongside poached or scrambled eggs on whole-grain bread. High-quality protein may be found in eggs, and avocados offer healthful fats and a creamy texture.

5. Yoghurt Salad:
Arrange granola, sliced kiwis, and honey drizzled over low-fat yogurt. Probiotics, fiber, and vitamins are combined in this parfait to create a tasty and nourishing breakfast.

Advice: Tailor these concepts to your tastes and tolerance. If you want to feel full all morning, try to maintain a healthy ratio of protein, fiber, and healthy fats.

Lunch and Dinner Suggestions

Lunch and dinner are opportunities to add a touch of culinary harmony to your day — meals that support your Crohn's disease journey while also providing nourishment. The following lunch and dinner ideas have been created with your wellbeing in mind:

1. Salad with Grilled Chicken:
Grilled chicken breast with cucumber, cherry tomatoes, and mixed greens on top. For a light and refreshing option, squeeze in some lemon and drizzle with olive oil.

2. Pilaf of Quinoa and Salmon:
Baked fish topped with chopped peas and bell peppers and served over quinoa pilaf. Omega-3 fatty acids are found in salmon, and protein and fiber are added in quinoa.

3. Plant-Based Stir-Fry:
Tempeh or tofu stir-fried with a vibrant mix of low-residue veggies, such as bell peppers, carrots, and zucchini. Serve over noodles or white rice for a filling plant-based meal.

4. Sweet potato with turkey skewers:
Skewers with sweet potato cubes and lean turkey slices alternately cooked to perfection. This recipe provides long-lasting energy by balancing protein and complex carbohydrates.

5. Curry with eggplant and chickpeas:
Simmered aubergine and chickpeas with a flavorful curry sauce, accompanied by basmati rice. This plant-based protein and fiber-rich vegetarian option is available.

Try varying the seasoning and cooking techniques to see what works best for your palate and digestive system. For a well-rounded lunch, concentrate on including a range of nutrients.

Snacks for Sustained Energy:

Snacks are essential for sustaining long-term energy levels, particularly for people with Crohn's disease. These are a few clever and filling snack suggestions to keep you going throughout the day:

1) Mixed Berries with Greek Yogurt:
Greek yogurt with reduced fat served with a few fresh berries. Probiotics, antioxidants, and protein are all present in this snack.

2) Banana slices with almond butter:
Rice cakes or whole-grain crackers with banana slices and almond butter on top. A delicious blend of fiber, natural sweetness, and good fats.

3) Personalized Trail Mix:
A combination of dried fruits, seeds, and nuts (walnuts, almonds). Tailor the mixture to your tastes, making sure that the right amounts of healthy fats and protein are included.

4) Sticks of vegetables with hummus:

Carrots, cucumbers, and bell peppers are crunchy vegetable sticks that are served with hummus on the side. Hummus gives this filling snack more taste and protein.

5)   Hard-Boiled Eggs:
Hard-boiled eggs seasoned with a dash of pepper and salt. Eggs are a convenient way to get important nutrients and high-quality protein.

<u>Advice</u>: Pay attention to your body's hunger signals and select nutrient-dense foods. Limit the amount you eat to prevent overtaxing your digestive system.

Three main considerations went into creating these meal and snack ideas: flavor, digestibility, and nutrition. As always, the secret is to experiment, figure out what suits you best, and enjoy the process of learning which meals are in harmony with your health.

CHAPTER 5

EXPERT ADVICE AND PROFESSIONAL GUIDANCE

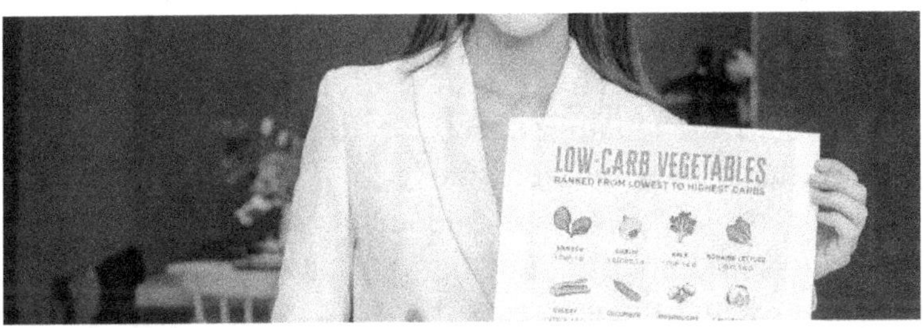

Setting out on a path to well-being needs not only willpower but also the direction of knowledgeable professionals who know their way around the complex world of diet and health. We explore the knowledge offered by eminent dietitians, nutritionists, and medical specialists in this chapter. Think of this as your culinary journey's compass, guiding you towards wise decisions and environmentally friendly methods.

Working Together with a Registered Dietitian: A Tailored Strategy

A "one-size-fits-all" approach to Crohn's disease management is insufficient. Your allies in creating a customized and successful nutrition plan are registered dietitians (RDs). Their ability to customize dietary suggestions to your unique situation while taking into account things like lifestyle, nutritional deficits, and the intensity of your symptoms can have a significant impact on your recovery.

To guarantee expert advice, look for a licenced dietician with gastrointestinal health experience.

Nutritional Therapies: Combining Healing with Science
By using food as medicine, nutritional therapies provide novel methods of treating Crohn's disease symptoms. These treatments, which include specific carbohydrate diets (SCD) and exclusive enteral nutrition (EEN), are supported by scientific research and are intended to minimize nutrient absorption, promote gut healing, and lessen inflammation. Speaking with medical experts who are knowledgeable about these methods can pave the way for a more individualized and comprehensive approach to nutrition management.

Advice: Before beginning any nutritional therapy regimen, make sure to speak with your healthcare provider to make sure it will meet your unique needs.

Synergy Between Medication and Nutrition

Medication is an essential part of the toolkit for treating Crohn's disease since it helps control inflammation and symptoms. Combining medication with well-planned eating habits results in a synergistic strategy. Work together with your nutritionist and healthcare provider to make sure that your diet supports your medication regimen and promotes overall health and optimal symptom control.

Advice: Be honest with your medical staff about your food preferences and any worries you may have about how certain medications may interact with certain foods.

Ways of Living: Exceeding the Plate

Well-being is a multifaceted concept that is influenced by lifestyle decisions and goes beyond what is placed on your plate. Getting enough sleep, controlling stress, and engaging in regular exercise all play a big part in controlling Crohn's disease symptoms. Your nutritionist can assist you in implementing lifestyle changes that support your health objectives and encourage a thorough and long-term approach to wellbeing.

Advice: To support your nutritional efforts, give self-care activities like mindfulness and enough sleep first priority.

Your Crohn's disease journey is dynamic, characterized by shifts in dietary requirements, lifestyle, and symptoms. Consistent follow-ups with your dietitian and medical team guarantee continued supervision and assistance. These partnerships enable you to modify your diet so that it progresses with you towards your goal of optimum health.

Advice: Maintain a health journal to document symptoms, dietary modifications, and lifestyle choices. This will help you and your healthcare team have productive conversations.

As you take in the knowledge from this chapter, think of it as a base upon which to construct your own customized nutrition and wellness strategy. Recall that your path is distinct, and that every decision you make can lead to a healthier, more robust version of yourself with the correct direction. To the science and art of managing Crohn's disease under professional supervision: enjoy the ride.

CHAPTER 6

TALES OF TRIUMPH

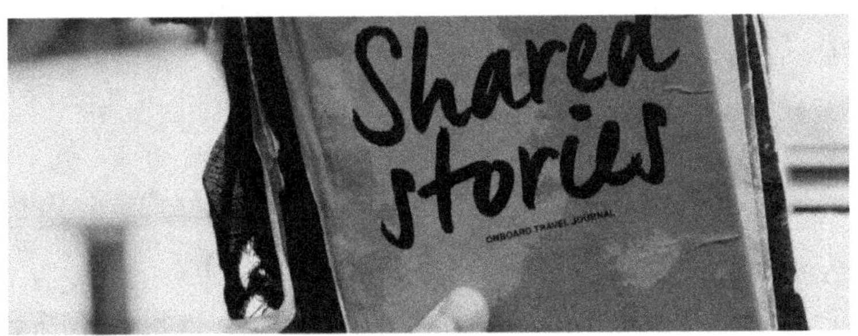

Welcome to Chapter 6 of "Crohn's Disease Food List." We explore a selection of narratives in these pages that demonstrate the transforming potential of healthy decisions. These are not merely triumph stories; they are accounts of people who set out on a quest to recover their well-being, equipped with the knowledge found in these chapters. Let the stories within guide you as you turn the pages, illuminating the significant relationship between resilience, food, and overcoming Crohn's disease obstacles.

Success Stories through Diet

Tales of success pop up in the fabric of Crohn's disease care, like rays of hope, demonstrating the life-changing potential of a thoughtfully planned diet. Here, we feature motivational testimonies from people who took the "Crohn's Disease Food List" as a guide and started on their path to wellness.

Meet Sarah: Disclosing Vitality via Taste Selections

Before Sarah adopted the Crohn's-friendly diet described in our book, her path with Crohn's disease was a maze of difficulties. Sarah started including nutrient-dense foods, putting balance and variety first despite her initial skepticism. Sarah experienced a significant change as the weeks passed into months: her energy increased and the frequency of flare-ups decreased. Sarah says, "My body seems to have found its beat." I'm living with Crohn's disease, not simply surviving it."

John's Gourmet Renaissance: A Healing Feast

John loved to eat and was worried that having Crohn's would make him less of a foodie. Still, a gastronomic renaissance was spurred by our book's emphasis on thoughtful preparation and well-balanced choices. John found that by experimenting with low-residue cooking methods and using gut-friendly ingredients, his digestive discomfort significantly decreased in addition to his newfound love for cooking. His kitchen evolved into a nurturing sanctuary, demonstrating the harmonious coexistence of taste and health.

Grace's Snack Discovery

Grace believed that the art of nibbling held the key to long-lasting energy and easy digestion. Equipped with the book's recommended snacks, Grace waved goodbye to energy slumps and welcomed foods that nourished rather than taxed her stomach. "Snacking became an excitement of trying new amazing combinations," she recalls. Who thought that something as basic as berry yogurt could have such a profound effect?"

James's Path to Remission: A Healing Symphony

Before he committed to the Crohn's-friendly meal plans, James's experience with Crohn's disease had been characterized by ups and downs. James saw a long-lasting remission by including nutrient-dense grains, lean proteins, and gut-soothing options. His narrative serves as evidence of the life-changing power of purposefully preparing meals and surrendering to the cadence of a healing symphony.

These triumphant tales demonstrate the concrete influence that deliberate dietary selections, as delineated in the "Crohn's Disease Food List," can yield on those managing Crohn's disease. Every narrative honors tenacity, energy, and the significant relationship between health and the plate. Let these stories encourage and direct you on your path towards a future full of sustenance, happiness, and victory over Crohn's disease obstacles as you go out on your own.

CHAPTER 7

PRACTICAL TIPS FOR EVERYDAY LIVING

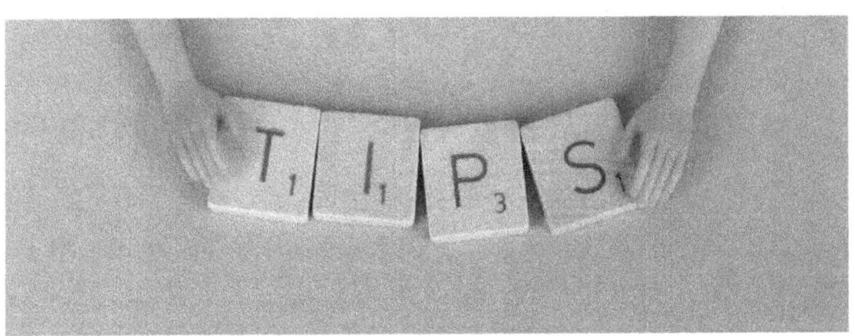

The dining room table is just one part of the stage in the symphony of managing Crohn's disease. "Crohn's Disease Food List" provides a comprehensive guidance that goes beyond food in Chapter 7, which offers a plethora of useful advice for daily living. These insights are meant to help you navigate the complexities of everyday life with resilience, balance, and well-being. They are derived from the knowledge of nutritionists and healthcare professionals.

1. Mindful Eating:

The technique of mindful eating, which goes beyond simply eating to become a life-changing experience, is fundamental to daily life. You may develop a healthy connection with food by taking your time, enjoying every meal, and being aware of your body's signals of hunger and fullness. This mindful technique strengthens the bond between the body and mind while also improving digestion.

Tip: To completely enjoy the sensory experience of your meals, create a calm and distraction-free dining setting.

2. Hydration Habits

Being well hydrated is essential for overall health, especially for people with Crohn's disease. Consuming enough fluids promotes healthy digestion, facilitates the absorption of nutrients, and guards against side effects like constipation. Make it a habit to stay hydrated by trying out different drinks like herbal teas, healthy broths, and water.

Tip: To guarantee constant fluid intake throughout the day, carry a reusable water bottle and set hydration goals.*

3. Techniques for Stress Management

One powerful factor affecting intestinal health is stress. It's critical to include stress-reduction techniques into your everyday activities. Discovering your own unique rhythm of quiet, whether via mindfulness exercises, deep breathing techniques, or joy-filled hobbies, greatly enhances the health of your body and mind.

Tip: Set aside some time every day for a stress-relieving activity that you enjoy doing, such as meditation, hiking, or creative endeavors.

4. Hygiene of Sleep

A valuable ally in the quest of general health is restful sleep. Restorative nights are facilitated by creating a regular sleep schedule, making the most of your sleeping environment, and adhering to proper sleep hygiene. Not only does getting enough sleep aid in physical recuperation, but it also enhances resilience and mood.

Tip: Make your room comfortable for sleeping by keeping the temperature at a reasonable level, lowering the lights, and limiting screen time before bed.

5. Exercise as Medicine

Engaging in physical activity is a powerful remedy for overall health, providing advantages not only for the physical body but also for the cerebral and emotional domains. Make your workout regimen unique to your tastes and capabilities by selecting enjoyable activities that support your health objectives. Frequent movement promotes general vigor, eases tension, and aids with digestion.

Tip: See what resonates with you by trying out different hobbies, such as yoga, strength training, or leisurely walks.

6. Social Support Networks

It takes a team to navigate Crohn's disease obstacles. Create a network of friends, family, and medical experts who are committed to your well-being and who understand it. Emotional resilience is enhanced by open communication, shared experiences, and a feeling of community, which also acts as a safety net in trying times.

Tip: To meet people who have gone through similar things, join support groups online or in person.

This chapter covers more ground than just diet; it covers the fabric of daily existence. By incorporating these useful suggestions into your daily routine, you may strengthen your ability to manage Crohn's disease and cultivate a way of life that values overall well-being. As you adopt these habits, allow every decision you make to become a note in your life's harmonic symphony. May every day be a fulfilling celebration dedicated to the art and science of living well with Crohn's disease!

CHAPTER 8

NAVIGATING GROCERY SHOPPING

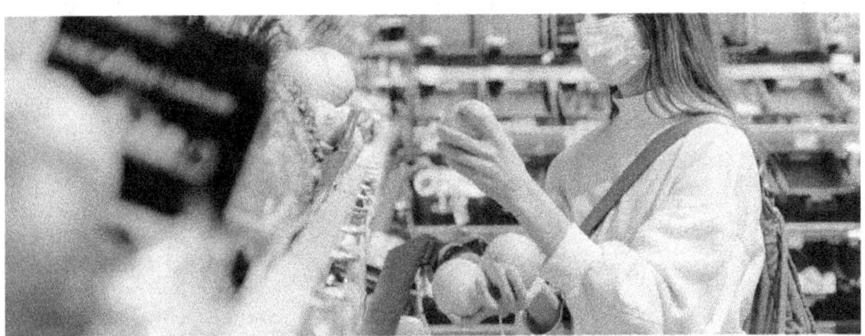

Greetings from Chapter 8, where we address the day-to-day practicalities of living with Crohn's disease. This section delves into the skill of food shopping, which is a vital component of creating a supportive and healthy environment for your health.

Making a Crohn's-Friendly Shopping List

Shopping for groceries is like the overture to your cooking concert, and making a grocery list that is Crohn's friendly is like writing a song of health. Start by determining the staple foods that provide the bulk of your meals and are high in nutrients and easily absorbed. In a harmonious and nourishing ensemble, fresh fruit, lean proteins, whole grains, and gut-friendly snacks take center stage.

<u>**Advice**</u>: To make grocery shopping easier, plan your meals for the coming week and make a thorough list of everything you need.

Getting Around the Grocery Store

It can be intimidating to navigate the grocery store aisles, but with the right strategy, it can be a smooth and uplifting experience. The following advice will help you:

1. **Shop the Periphery**: Pay attention to the areas around the produce, lean meats, and dairy products, as these are usually found there. This aids in giving whole, unprocessed foods first priority.
2.
2. **Carefully read the labels:**Spend some time reading food labels, focusing on the nutritional information and ingredients. Select goods that fit your nutritional objectives and have the fewest additives, preservatives, and substances possible.

3. **Stock Up on Gut-Friendly Staples:** Make sure your cupboard is full of foods that are excellent for your gut, like easily digested proteins, low-residue grains, and nutritionally sound canned products.

4. **Accept Online Shopping:** Take into account online grocery delivery services, which let you make your list while lounging in your house. This offers a regulated setting for decision-making in addition to time savings.

<u>**Advice**</u>: Check out specialist or health food stores as they can have a greater selection of foods that are suitable for Crohn's disease sufferers.

Creating Convenient and Robust Meals

The foundation of an organized and effective life with Crohn's disease is meal preparation. You can ensure that nourishing options are always available while also streamlining your daily routine by setting aside time to prepare and portion meals in advance. Plan your meals, make an investment in high-quality storage containers, and relish the ease of having wholesome options close at hand.

Start with easy-to-make dishes that you can modify to make different meals every day of the week.

Eating Out with Crohn's Disease

Grocery shopping establishes the scene, but eating out creates fresh dynamics. Prepare yourself by learning how to read restaurant menus and making decisions that are in line with your health:

1. Examine Menus in Advance: Check out a restaurant's online menu before you go. This enables you to recognise Crohn's-friendly items and make decisions in advance.

2. Share Dietary Needs: Don't be afraid to let the restaurant personnel know what your dietary requirements are. Many places are happy to fulfill unique requests or make adjustments.

3. Select Easier Preparations: Go with easier culinary techniques like baking, steaming, or grilling. They frequently cause less harm to the digestive tract.

Exercise caution while determining portion sizes. In order to prevent overtaxing your digestive tract, think about splitting dishes or requesting a half-portion.

Advice: Make decisions that support your enjoyment and health objectives while concentrating on the fun of dining out and the social aspects of the occasion.

We've broken down the ins and outs of grocery shopping and eating out in this chapter, arming you with the knowledge and skills to confidently tackle these common obstacles. Let every decision you make as you incorporate these techniques into your everyday activities become a note in the harmony of your wellbeing. To the skill and science of managing day-to-day living with Crohn's disease: may every encounter be a fulfilling joy!

Sample Crohn's-Friendly Meal Plan

Starting a Crohn's disease management path means preparing meals that are high in digestibility, nutrient density, and gut-friendly options. This meal plan sample acts as a model, providing a resilient and nourishing day that adheres to the guidelines provided in the "Crohn's Disease Food List."

MEAL PLAN #1

I. Breakfast: Quinoa Breakfast Bowl

-
- One cup of cooked quinoa
- One medium banana, cut into slices
- One spoonful of chia seeds
- half cup of Greek yogurt

Instructions: Add quinoa, chia seeds, banana slices, and Greek yogurt on top. This breakfast offers a combination of probiotics, fiber, and protein.

II. Mid-Morning Snack: Almond Butter and Apple Slices

- Two tsp almond butter
- One medium apple, cut into slices

Instructions: For a filling snack high in good fats and natural sweetness, spread almond butter on apple slices.

III. Lunch: Grilled Chicken Salad

- 4 ounces of grilled, sliced chicken breast
- mixed greens, including kale, spinach and rocket
- Half a cucumber, cut, and cherry tomatoes with 1 tablespoon of olive oil
- Lemon juice as a dressing

Instructions: Combine cucumber, tomatoes, grilled chicken, and mixed greens to make the salad. For a light and revitalizing meal, drizzle with olive oil and lemon juice.

IV. Afternoon Snack: Greek Yogurt with Berries

- half cup of Greek yogurt
- Berries in combination (strawberries, blueberries)

Instructions: For a high-protein and antioxidant snack, top Greek yogurt with a handful of mixed berries.

V. Dinner: Salmon and Quinoa Pilaf

- Six ounces of baked salmon
- One cup of cooked quinoa
- Vegetable mixture (peas, bell peppers)
- One tablespoon of olive oil

Instructions: Bake the fish and serve it with mixed vegetables and quinoa pilaf. For a supper of nutrient-dense cereals and omega-3 fatty acids, drizzle with olive oil.

VI. Evening Snack: Hard-Boiled Eggs

- Two eggs, hard-boiled
- A dash of pepper and salt

Instructions: For a quick and high-protein evening snack, season hard-boiled eggs with salt and pepper.

VII. Hydration Throughout the Day:

- Drink water at regular intervals during the day.
- For variation, try adding infused water or herbal teas.

<u>Notes</u>: Lean proteins, good fats, and complex carbohydrates are among the macronutrients that are balanced in this sample meal plan. In order to support your digestive health and general well-being, it places an emphasis on foods that are readily digested and high in nutrients. Don't forget to modify this plan to suit your own nutritional requirements, tolerances, and preferences. For individualized guidance, speak with a nutritionist or other medical professional.

SAMPLE MEAL PLAN #2

This alternative sample complies with the guidelines provided in the "Crohn's Disease Food List" and offers a range of flavors and textures. Please feel free to alter according to your dietary requirements, tolerances, and preferences.

I. Smoothie Bowl Delight for breakfast

- One cup of spinach leaves
- half of a frozen banana
- Half a cup of frozen berries (raspberries and blueberries)
- One spoonful of chia seeds
- 1/2 cup almond milk or lactose-free yogurt.

Instructions: Smoothly blend spinach, banana, chia seeds, berries, and almond or yogurt milk. For a nutrient-dense breakfast, top with sliced strawberries and granola.

II. Mid-Morning Snack: Rice Cake with Avocado

- Two cakes of rice
- 1/2 mashed, ripe avocado
- A pinch of black pepper and sea salt.

Instructions: Top rice cakes with mashed avocado and sprinkle with salt and pepper. A filling snack full of fiber and good fats.

III. Lunch: Quinoa and Veggie Stuffed Peppers

- Two peppers, cut in half
- One cup of cooked quinoa
- mixed veggies, including spinach, cherry tomatoes and zucchini
- 4 oz of ground tofu or turkey
- One tablespoon of olive oil.

Instructions: In olive oil, sauté mixed vegetables and ground tofu or turkey. Blend with the cooked quinoa and press into the halves of bell peppers. Bake peppers until they are soft for a tasty, well-rounded meal.

IV. Snack in the afternoon: veggie sticks and hummus

- 1/2 cup hummus
- Assorted vegetable sticks (carrots, cucumber, bell peppers)

Instructions: Dip your vegetable sticks into hummus for a crunchy and satisfying snack providing you plant-based protein and fiber.

V. Dinner: Baked Cod with Sweet Potato Mash

- Six-ounce baked cod filet
- Boil and mash one medium sweet potato
- Steam-cooked broccoli
- slices of lemon as a garnish.

Instructions: Serve steamed broccoli alongside mashed sweet potatoes and baked cod with a squeeze of lemon. A delicious supper high in complex carbohydrates and lean protein.

VI. Snack in the evening: Dried fruits and mixed nuts

- 1/4 cup of mixed nuts (walnuts and almonds)
- 1/4 cup of dried fruit (cranberries, apricots).

Instructions: For a filling and energizing evening snack, blend your own nuts and dried fruits.

VII. Staying Hydrated During the Day:

Drink water, herbal teas, or water that has been infused with cucumber or mint slices.

Notes: To accommodate a range of tastes and interests, this alternative meal plan offers a varied assortment of nutrient-dense meals.

Modify serving sizes according to your needs; for individualized advice, speak with a dietician or healthcare provider.

CONCLUSION

We celebrate the completion of a journey as you approach the last pages of the "Crohn's Disease Food List"—a journey towards empowerment, resilience, and sustenance. You deserve praise for your dedication to controlling Crohn's disease, and these chapters include a wealth of information, wisdom, and useful tools to help you get well.

You've learned the art of creating meals that flow in unison with the distinct beat of your body from the symphony of nutritional options. Every page has been a step closer to a happier and more empowered existence, from the basics of Crohn's-friendly diet to the professional advice and useful hints for daily living.

You Are in Control: Keep in mind that no two journeys are alike, and with the insights in this book, you can design the life you want. You have the brush to create a resilient canvas, the pen to write stories of success, and the conductor's baton to create a vibrant symphony. Accept that you have the ability to make decisions that are in harmony with your mind, body, and spirit.

You are not an isolated thread in the fabric of wellness. Beside you is a network of others who have traveled similar paths as well as medical professionals and nutritionists. Seek out assistance, talk to others about your experiences, and take courage from the combined knowledge of those who have experienced both the struggles and triumphs of living with Crohn's disease.

As you put the ideas in this book into practice, focus on making progress rather than perfection. Every conscious decision, every healthy meal, and every stride in the direction of wellbeing is a victory. Your path is made up of a patchwork of tiny triumphs that together create a bright image of your strong, independent life.

This is not the end; rather, it is the start of a new chapter in which you will continue to inspire others and live your life on your terms. Savor every taste, appreciate how easy it is to prepare healthy meals, and feel empowered to make decisions that support your health objectives.

Let this book be your traveling partner on this inspiring voyage, to sum up. I hope it can be used as a guide, an inspiration, and a reminder to prioritize and take care of your well-being. Your contentment, fortitude, and energy are paramount, and with the wisdom acquired, you hold the keys to opening doors to a future full of strength, hope, and well-earned happiness.

May every day be an ode to the amazing person you are!

<u>My Little Request</u>

Thank You For Reading This Book!
I really appreciate all of your feedback and
I love to hear what you have to say.

Please take 1 minute now to leave a helpful 5-Star
review on Amazon if you enjoyed the book.
Thanks so much!
Bell Quintana

NOTES

(For Your Favorite Recipes or Notes)

Attribution

All images used in this book were downloaded from *pixabay.com* and *pexels.com*.